Sex Esteem

ASHA BIANCA

Definition of Sex Esteem - finding our esteem/identity
outside of God's truth of who we are.

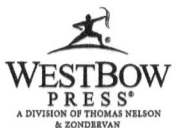

WESTBOW
PRESS®
A DIVISION OF THOMAS NELSON
& ZONDERVAN

WestBow Press books may be ordered through booksellers or by contacting:

WestBow Press
A Division of Thomas Nelson & Zondervan
1663 Liberty Drive
Bloomington, IN 47403
www.westbowpress.com
1 (866) 928-1240

Illustrations by Kali Bradford

ISBN: 978-1-5127-3691-5 (sc)

Print information available on the last page.

WestBow Press rev. date: 4/28/2016

dedicated to those who remind me of my identity, heart and tingles.

Papa Maza for hours in the car speaking truth. Shawn, Larry, Chris, Shane for over twenty years of teaching. Women who have become soul sisters loving me inside and out, bringing me coffee, hiking year after year arm in arm, praying for me and wholly investing in me, my daughter and all my youth girls for inspiring me to be a good role model - too many to name but those closest to me, know who they are. God who loves me the most and best.

Contents

Who Sex Esteem is for?

God has a pretty funny sense of humor. Its January 2016 and I am holed up in my favorite cottage writing this book, a book that has been in my head for years, going on ten years actually. At this current moment, I am being pursued by someone who thinks I hung the moon. I have not had sex with this someone. I am wrestling with a new frontier as a youth leader of many years who now is getting to practice what I have preached through living pure, not only but primarily abstaining from sex. I find this comical because I am writing a book on Sex Esteem while wrestling with what that truly means. I love how God takes us right to the edge so our continual reliance is on Him not us. So let's roll, not literally.

I spent years finding my identity through the wrong channels, pick one and there will be a story about it…..sex, work, motherhood, marriage, friendship…..the list goes on. I am now at a place where I can see the balance between being a woman of God and being a woman who understands her passion, worth and value. It is a beautiful landing place.

Passion has always been part of my DNA. During my Christian walk it has been ok to be passionate about God, children, missions, youth and things that are generally "accepted" as the things good Christians are passionate about.

The rub, as our awesome Shakespeare would say, is that today's world has not allowed us to be passionate about the sensual things in life. We have a whole side of us that is very sensual and wired by God that way. We have done a lousy job encouraging married couples to have more sex than anyone and it seems that the hottest, wildest worlds are far from the creator who actually created this pleasure in the first place. We have lots of sex before marriage and then little to none after. We have it backwards.

This book is intended for individuals navigating several different stages of their lives. These are the beautiful people who I had in mind when God laid this story on my heart. I am not a scholar, I am a woman who is trying to share her truths of finding her esteem in the wrong places verses the right truths.

I am writing this from a place of love, not judgement, as we know from **Romans 8:1, There is no condemnation for those who belong to Christ Jesus.** This is a truth, and for too long, many of us have believed untruths about ourselves. We will tackle these together. One of the last chapters of Sex Esteem is actually titled Truth.

For the Girls -

Sex Esteem is for girls just entering their teens where the pressure to be a certain way is monumental. For middle school girls this is the first time in their life that their bodies become more the focus than their beings. This is a tricky time to say the least.

I remember that first moment when I was self conscious about going swimming in my tank and undies, when the same activity had not caused a moment of pause previously. This change is heavy to navigate and without the right truths and support in place can shake a young girl's self. This was the case for me.

Middle school ages are a fork in the road where we choose what kind of activities we will engage in, talking, touching, thinking, etc. For many of us, this happens quite early in life, for others it is later, either way these are worlds that become more real than ever before during these ages.

I currently serve as a youth leader to freshman and sophomore girls. Previously I led middle school girls, I have seen girls who make decisions about how they will interact to obtain sex esteem at the cost of their true esteem at this stage in life that affect them for years to come. I have been one of those girls. Having pregnancy scares in 7th grade is something no girl should have to walk through. Wondering when "he" will call, what "he" will send/text next, how far will "he" go removes a place of innocence from the world of adolescence that then is desperately longing to be fixed.

I don't think we were intended to deal with these types of heavy topics right when we are just beginning to learn about these beautiful feelings that God has wired us with. Many of the self-harm issues that our youth face today result from this premature exposure, this book is primarily written for women but men have their equal weighty counters. I write from my experience as a woman, who didn't navigate this issue well, then by the grace of God, has learned who to turn to for my esteem, who I am without a man, what I was bought with and how much I am worth.

Also, I have seen girls who resolve to be themselves, regardless of the attention being thrust on them. These girls are few and far between but I must confide in you, they are my heroes. To know yourself and who you are in God as not to be shaken makes me in awe of them. For families who create this type of stability from a young woman's self-worth, I respect you tremendously. God has placed on my heart a need to support girls through this time period. Thankful for my experiences both good and place that are being used to lessen pain, and gain ground.

Guidelines such as the below list can be extremely helpful before you are learning how to navigate these new feelings, so you can keep your head and your values in check:

Modesty is beautiful.

Most people do not marry their first loves, some do but most don't.

A person is very different in their teens than in their twenties. Know yourself and allow yourself to grow until you are fully yourself. Its very hard to be with someone, when you aren't certain who you are yet. Not to mention to choose the right someone.

Even though others may not know, what you do, text, type, say all have an impact on you.

Pay attention to how they treat you, always.

Talk with your parents or a trusted mentor openly and honestly.

Secrets leave scars on the inside.

Know who God says you are before listening to who anyone else says you are.

Take a couple minutes and ask yourself, "how will I feel about myself after I say/write/do this?"

Breathe, be aware, have clean fun and don't beat yourself up.

Keep yourself safe, magic needs to be protected. You are righteous magic.

Next for the Wild Women -

Oh do I have a heart for you, and I'm not the only one. I got an early start to my wild women days before I even was a woman. God has a heart for wild women also.

When researching various words come to mind for the word wild, the dictionary defines wild as living in a state of nature; not tamed or domesticated. State of nature, which was created by God, isn't such a far cry from how I think of wild also. I have to say I love this word, wild. Say it slow and loud, beautiful! I love the way it is intended, I think of John the Baptist immediately, a wild passion for His King. I think of the way God shined His light through an extreme wild woman named Rahab, who according to the Book of Joshua, was a prostitute who lived in Jericho in the Promised Land and assisted the Israelites in capturing the city. Moments before she was used by God, she wasn't asked to clean-up her wild ways. Now I'm not a big fan of prostitution but I am a big fan of a God who meets us where we are and uses our real world experiences to change the world through us.

Part of me wishes I had a different story to tell about my first interactions with sex. I long for a story of waiting and being married and feeling protected in a way that only God can heal. However, because of my experiences, I can relate to youth who I coach through life in a way that I may not have been able to had I not had those experiences.

I sit squarely with the truth of this verse, **Romans 8:28, And we know that in all things God works for the good of those who love him, who have been called according to his purpose.** To me, this means that while God would like me to be protected from certain elements of this world, he doesn't stop using me because I have made poor choices in the past. He can turn every single trash choice into a treasure in the life of someone who needs encouragement.

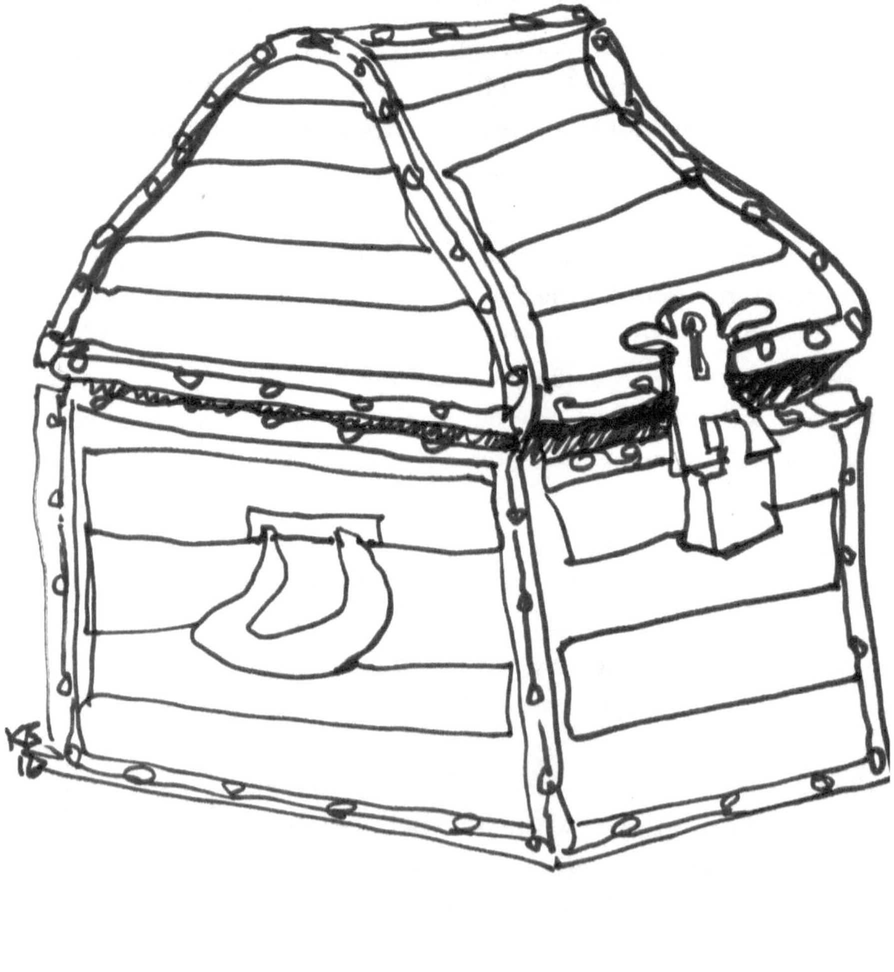

Courage comes from surviving through experiences. The actual word encourage means to impart courage into another. We can infuse courage into others by shining God's light into a world that desperately needs it. We can be bold enough to talk about the topics that most people don't talk about, dive into the feelings that God has wired us with instead of putting our hands up in the face of people wrestling with these feelings and imply that just say no, is as easy as it sounds.

So this mention is for those women who were promiscuous in ways that stole your innocence, this book is for you. I want you to spend extra time in the truth chapter. There is an enemy who wants nothing more than to render you useless for the kingdom because of choices in your past. The world is both enthralled by your being as wild as you can and then equally condemning once you have been. Some of the worst evil is from judgement that comes down in this area.

Truth allows you to know who you are and move forward because of it. You are a cherished daughter of the King. You are righteous, loved and worthy.

Guidelines such the below list can be extremely helpful when you want to change the way you have operated in your past, so you can keep your head and your values in check:

> Stop allowing any bad memories or experiences in your head.

> If you can't, see a counselor and pray.

> You are not your past, remember this.

> You are in a battle and your passion is an awesome gift for advancing the Kingdom when it is in His will.

> He either didn't know better or didn't love you that much, if he went against God's plan for how it could be best.

You are worth a wait, no matter how long that wait is, for the right partner.

Say no to shame.

No guilt just grace.

Now for the Wife

Ok, this has been a part of this book that I am pretty excited about. You get to have sex with your husband anytime you want, yes anytime! Guess what, the silly notion that sex is only for men is bologna, sex is as much for you as it is for your husband.

Sex was created by God to be the glue of your marriage. When was the last time you tried to do a craft that called for glue with out glue, how'd that work? Not so well, in my experience. You are allowed to be sexy and a woman of your husband's dreams.

I understand there are women who think holding out and using sex as a carrot is a way to feed the idol of control, stop. You are called to be a partner of your husband. Your body is his and his is yours, enjoy it. Sex in marriage with your life partner is good, enjoy every minute!

My recommendation for you is have sex at least everyday whether you "feel" like it or not. You'll have to visit the gym less and your marriage will be leveraging the glue that God provided. I recognize there will be days when it just doesn't happen, oh well, make the next day even better. Take back your marriage bed and make each other's dreams come true together.

Side bar - one of the saddest moments after I filed for divorce and the word got out was women bringing their complaints about their husbands to me. These complaints were not severe, they weren't adultery or abuse, they weren't fear or misconduct. They were complaints. My recommendations to each of them was the same, starting today have sex with your husband every day for the next month and then let me know how it goes.

Guidelines such the below list can be extremely helpful before you complain about your husband, so you can keep your head and your values in check:

Pray for him and your heart from him.

Remember he has physical needs too, feed them.

Don't complain. Its unattractive.

Be Kind. Its attractive.

Make time for just you two.

Support him.

Praise publicly, give him your input, if it conflicts with his, as privately as possible.

Know what he likes, do it.

Talking on the phone for long periods of time with a girlfriend, mother, etc. is a turn-off.

Wear lingerie and lots of it.

Remember to pamper his mind, spirit and body.

Think less of what you are getting out of the marriage and focus on giving.

Tell him, and only him when he is missing the mark. Bring in a counselor if needed.

Only seek marriage advice from those who share your beliefs on marriage.

Lastly for the Single Searcher/Divorcee/Widow/Girlfriend

I have a new found respect for you, I am currently in this category. Whether you have always been single, have been through a divorce or are a widow, this is a new world to navigate.

During this phase when it comes to sex, I'll write from the place I am at, which is no sex before marriage. Upon seeking counsel in this area, my pastor told a gentleman admirer who was asking what he and his girlfriend can do, "you know what you can't do, right." The pastor went on to say that they needed to talk about how far was too far and make sure to error on the side of conservative touch both for hormone control and to align with God's word of not even a "hint" of immorality. This is solid advice.

Too often we want to push the limits of what we "can" do, instead of letting the spirit lead and putting the proper proactive measures in place.

Reminders such as the below list can be extremely helpful before you are in a moment of let's just say fogged windows, so you can keep your head and your values in check:

Don't be alone for overlong time periods in private places. This is a tricky one for me because I love to hike, luckily where I hike, the temperature is rarely above 10 degrees for 6 months out of the year, so I have plenty of clothes on.

If one chooses to drink, don't drink more than you are able to maintain your good judgement.

Compromising is a slippery slope.

If drinking always leads to poor choices, don't drink.

This isn't brain surgery, you know your hot buttons so avoid those.

If you are dating someone, make sure they very clearly understand what is and isn't acceptable. As my friend said, "you don't want to ruin a beautiful adventure with an awkward moment."

Share about the person, their texts, red flags you may be feeling, good stuff, not so good stuff with your confidants.

Talk about what you will and won't do early and often. Your body is in fact your temple and it deserves an incredible amount of respect.

Its more difficult to make good decisions late at night. Be aware of what your plans will be after the party/date, etc.

Be careful while dancing not to send the wrong message to the wrong person.

Anything you need a blanket to cover up, is not a good idea.

Think of anything you type and say as being broadcasted. This one I have to remind myself of regularly!

Be more covered than you'd like to be in any water. Ideally a one piece with shirt/shorts. There's just something about water.

If the suitor has children, spend a lot of time with them, they will naturally keep you in check.

If you aren't able to talk, even uncomfortably, with that special him or her about something when it comes to your body, you may not be ready to be considering it or be in a relationship.

When you are being "courted" meaning pursued or someone is interested in you, it is the best they generally will ever treat you, remember this.

If the possible suitor has an objective to your limits, guess what he just saved you a ton of heart ache and time spent dressing up. Say a kind goodbye to him and be glad you have standards. This I've found to be the most efficient way to be true to my values.

I do have several friends who believe in sex outside of marriage and I talk with them regularly to ensure I understand both sides of the choice.

Although, I defer to the bible as a black and white matter here, understanding the dominate cultural norms is important. The dominate cultural norm in today's world, is to have sex before marriage. To deny the huge influence the world has on sex would be to live under a rock and I like light.

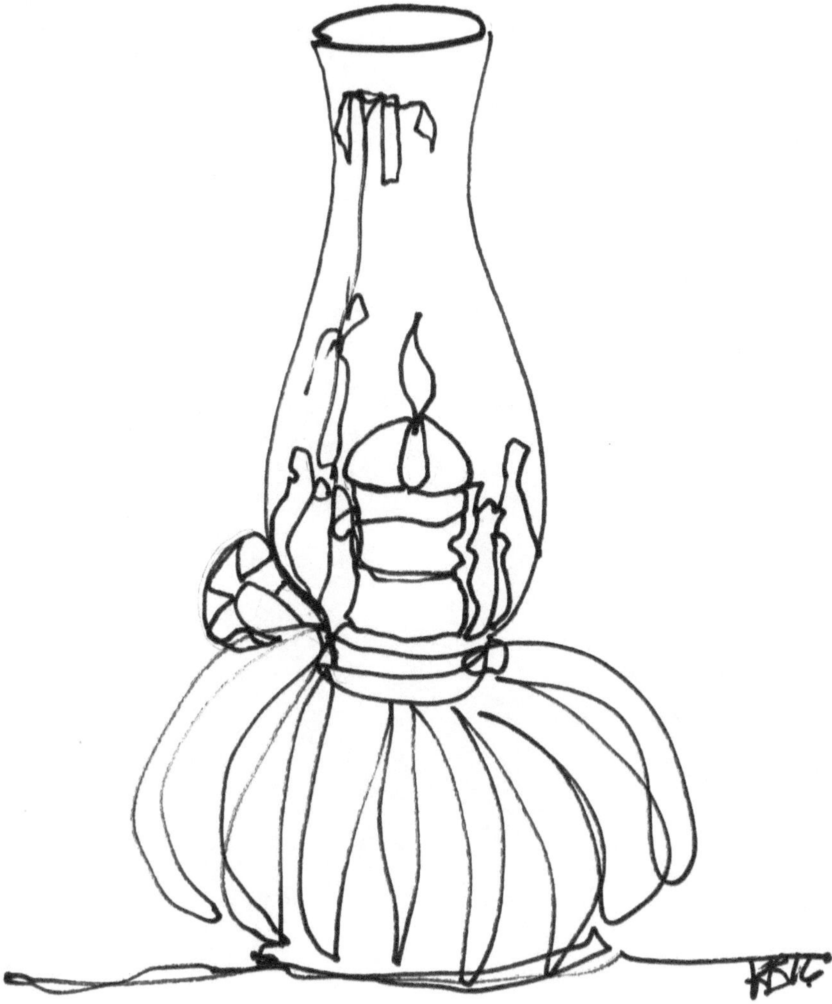

What is that feeling?

Ok so now that we know who this book, Sex Esteem, is written for, let's dive into why we have this dilemma of finding our esteem in areas that are not who we foundational are in Christ, specifically seeking the approval of the opposite sex for attention that is intended to come from our Creator.

Let's start with the beautiful story of the gospel, beginning in **Genesis 1:27 - So God created mankind in his own image, in the image of God he created them; male and female he created them.**

We each were created in God's own image, flawless and completely full in power. He delighted in us and created us without sin. My favorite definition of sin is that which separates us from God. The reason I like this definition is it is true to the equalizing of all sins as well as removing the condemning word of shame that so often accompanies definitions of sin.

God created us, He knows us more intimately than anyone else, He loves us more completely than anyone else. So the very thought of being farther than I could be from Him, is an interesting one to land on for a moment.

To draw a parallel, I live very far away from my closest loved ones. I work in a big girl job that brought me thousands of miles to a town I had never heard of seven years ago. I am a practical person and when given the option to move and continue with a secure job while raising two children, the option was fairly obvious. That said, it pains me to live far from those I love, truly pains me.

My dad is one of the closest people in the world to me relationally, yet he lives a minimum of two plane trips away from me. His health isn't the best, this can be quite a challenge when I need to be there for him. My daughter who brings me such delight every single day also lives a minimum of two plane rides away from me. My brother's entire family who sometimes feel like oxygen to me live on the completely opposite side of the country. I state these facts because where people are as it relates in proximity to you is important. Try as I might to be in my niece and nephew's life, it isn't feasible for me to catch their basketball games on a weekend. Time with them needs to be planned, purposeful and allotted. Learning to love long distance is a skill that can be refined but at the end of the day, being near both relationally and physically is critical for our strongest relationships.

This is true for our God as well, when we choose to spend time away from Him, it impacts our ability to hear and see Him in our lives. When we decide to put things that are not of Him before Him, He will allow us to.

This fact is terrifying, throughout the bible when people didn't want Jesus as part of their worlds, He would do one simple thing, He would leave. Take the rich man for instance who had a heart issue that Jesus wanted to talk about. Jesus wanted the rich man to understand that Jesus isn't just good, He is God. At the point where he had the decision to make God, the God of his own life, the man wasn't yet ready to give up his idols so Jesus let him have them and left him alone. This means that if you choose your idols, whatever they may be…gossip, lust, ideology of your image, social commitments, etc…He will let you have them instead of Him. These things will begin edging Him out of your life and you will have less impact in kingdom advancement and less joy through His strength.

Reading **1 Corinthian 6:17 - But whoever is united with the Lord is one with him in spirit.** We were designed to be with Jesus. In communion, without space, as one. When we choose other idols, we are choosing to create separation and space from how we were intended to live. His spirit is made to be our help-mate. I love this word, it is actually quite a powerful word in the bible. I think of power when I think of help-mate. The spirit actually lives in us and when leaned on becomes stronger because we were created to live in the spirit.

So how does this work practically. We were made with feelings, feeling of love, anger, sadness. We were made in the image of God in all His Glory. So what does this look like when I have the hots for some guy in my 4th period class or at work. Why do I get flush, why do I like when he tells me I'm beautiful. Its because we are creatures who want to find our value in something. We want to know we were made for a purpose and have worth.

The world is all too quick to provide that value and worth in a way that is counterfeit. We know that staying power for our identity only rests in God and who He says we are. That said, I think feelings sometimes get a bad wrap in Christian circles. I love that I can feel, it is one of my most powerful ways to advance the kingdom. Leaning into the spirit to direct the feelings is the critical piece.

I'll just come out and say it, I haven't ever been a fan of this next verse. Growing up the way I did without church and Jesus, my heart was always a near and dear piece of me. My dad even passed out little heart stickers to my friends in kindergarten. When I sign my books, I generally will draw a heart, it is my most used emoticon. I like heart, let's leave it at that. So you can see why this verse isn't one I will be stitching on a pillow soon. That said, I have come to gain a new respect for this verse.

Here it is, **Jeremiah 17:9 - The heart is deceitful above all things, and desperately sick; who can understand it?** The heart is definitely a mystery so I get that part, the deceitful part I am trusting God about. My heart and spirit seem to be very intertwined, just how I think about it. If I feel led to pay for a service man's dinner, give a special gift, edify with an encouraging word, I think about this as coming from my heart. When in all honesty, this is really coming from the spirit that lives in me. My heart is the same place that I might feel lust to go farther than I should, say something out of anger that would be better left unsaid. This is where I feel and feelings left unchecked without the spirit can absolutely be damaging.

This is why I believe God uses the word deceitful because feelings of the heart can be manipulating and confusing. If left to its own agenda without the spirit leading, the heart can think some pretty crazy feelings. I remember one day I was certain someone was the one. Now, I wasn't lining the one up against the clear instructions of who God says the one will look like, I was leaning on….yes, you guessed it, my heart. I love that God warns us to be on-guard and seek Him for conditions of the heart because left by itself, it is definitely squirrely.

For matters where we feel strongly about something, waiting, seeking, leaning into God is definitely what it is about. That impulsive response that so many of us have grown accustomed to from movies in particular, isn't necessarily the most healthy response in the majority of cases.

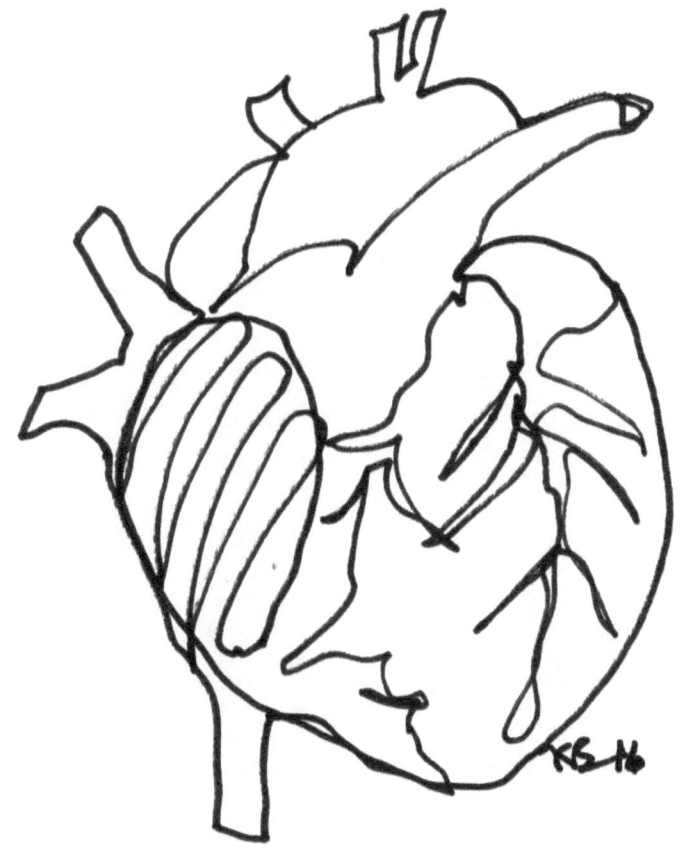

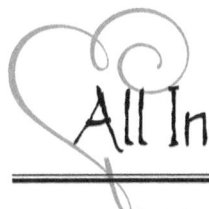

All In

Affection came to me fairly easily. Physical touch is one of my top two love languages, and I am Italian so needless to say, I have always been fairly huggy. I remember one particularly hot southern California day, I may have been ten years old at most when I wanted to snuggle up against my brother, after he said, "Osh, its too hot to snuggle." I then went over to my mom who had a similar response.

Touch to me is just how I am wired, I feel extremely connected with someone when I hold their hand, hug them, snug next to them. This is a part of me that I have grown to love. One of my friends who is a terrific mom but whose love language is not physical touch was complaining about how often her little ones cling on to her. She said, "they are always touching me". I was laughing thinking I so get that!

There is no doubt that each of us is wired differently, so early on I was very affectionate. I also had a boy best friend as a young one running around so there were a lot of innocent explorations when it came to touch. I had one scary experience that God protected me from. A stranger had come into the house and was about to touch my leg when I was about 8 and God woke me up and gave me the wisdom to say, "I have to use the restroom", when I returned he was gone and I felt safe again. God was always there for me even before I recognized Him.

I have never struggled with feeling like a child of God. Once at a soup house with my mom, I must have been 6 or 7 and they sang the song, He has the whole world in his hands. I sang along and felt like I truly knew who they sang about deep in my heart.

For someone who didn't attend church so to speak, I talked about white light a lot …white light is what I called God from early on, regularly.

I love this verse, **John 1:12 - Yet to all who did receive him, to those who believed in his name, he gave the right to become children of God.** What a beautiful family to be a part of. Everything good and innocent and beautiful I feel when I read this verse. God's way of showing us our own original beauty, a tender kind untainted beauty.

Commercially our world has turned this beauty into such an exploited thing. We as a culture have taken sweet young children, dressed them up and walked them out in shoes too high and lipstick too bright. I think this is why we long for old shows that show a simpler environment for our children, when it was safer and less exploited.

A time when if you wanted to give a girl attention, you'd have to get through her father, mother, any siblings, find where she lived, walk there and be pretty sure you knew what to say when you got there. The level of courage it took to actually talk with someone was off the charts. The level of courage today that it takes to give attention is seconds, I wouldn't even label the word courage next to it.

We have taken something previous called respect and lessened it to the inth degree. By lessening the impact of affection on our hearts and minds, by minimizing the impressions left by words and touch, we have hurt what it means to be a child of God.

Often when I am struggling loving a particular person whether at work or at home, I remember God loves them so incredibly much. I pray that He gives me eyes to see that person, the way God sees him or her. All of a sudden, He lifts the world view and lays a different view on me. This view is one that highlights their strengths, it highlights the purest form of them. The child of God in them.

When I was about 12, I became engrossed in attention from boys. Then, there wasn't texting or social media, it was more about looks, notes and secret rendezvous spots covered by some lie. It was easy to fall into and very soon my sole source of esteem was who liked me and how much. Now don't get me wrong, I still kept the other plates in the air....school, pets, friends...but it was a boy's look or word that carried a greater weight. I remember feeling tingles whenever he, whoever the particular he was, looked my way, sure it was superficial but it was also entrapping.

To say I went All In would be an understatement. I am committed to sin not getting a lot of air time, even in a book titled Sex Esteem. I try fiercely to remove anything that distracts from God and that is exactly what sin is, so I won't spend much time on details here but, just trust me when I say I was a teenage Rahab.

I gave myself away, I put myself in jeopardy, I didn't value myself unless there was a sparkle in some boys eyes looking at me. I was pretending to be a grown-up, while moment by moment emotionally I was losing ground. I think you could call my years from 12-19 lost years and in no way be wrong. I lost myself, I trusted people not worth my trust, I lowered my standards, I lost my true north, I lost my white light, I lost humility, I lost my innocence.

Writing about these experiences no longer holds any shame, regret or remorse for me. I am a new creation through Jesus. He has removed any stigma associated with this time of my life. The following verse shows that even though our heart reminds us of who we were, God reminds us of who we are in Him. **1 John 3:20 - For whenever our heart condemns us, God is greater than our heart, and he knows everything.** We are not choices we have made in the past, although we bear the consequences of those choices, we are a new creation every time we make the decision to recognize His sacrifice for us and let His spirit that lives in us lead.

When we know better we do better, when we have healthy support we won't tolerate unhealthy support, when we learn how important boundaries are we establish and adhere to them. I remember one year for halloween, I was 13 and I dressed-up in one of those adult french maid costumes, this is one visual memory that I associate summing up this time of my life. Otherwise I don't remember a ton about these years, I am thankful for God for that. I do remember though that all the esteem I had came from inappropriate attention, sex and the wrong kind of who I was as described by the world not truth.

If you are reading this and All In is your reality at the moment, my encouragement to you is to be very present about what you are choosing to do. Take extra time with every single decision, every word you text, every person you allow in your life.

With this way of life, there is a numbness that sets in fairly quickly when you are all in. This numbness becomes your new reality and the life you are living is no longer your own. Your acts are about others, your being and worth is about others. Your esteem hangs in the balance of what someone thinks about you, what they say to you, what they do to you. Your innocence, power and magic, as my brother would call it, is to be protected. It is something that once lost, is very difficult to find again.

At the time of falling all in, it can be intoxicating to think that someone's world even for a second is all about you. Believe me, this has way more to do with sheer hormones than anything else. Once the moment has passed, you are there with the next way to get your esteem up and a reminder that the world says you are not enough. This is a mistruth, you are enough by yourself however you chose to engage, you will never be more or less than the amazing person that Jesus died for so can stand justified and oh how I love this word....righteous.

So let's talk about righteous for a bit, it is such a beautiful concept and it unlike many of the other words this world has, is exclusively for us, children of God. We are righteous and beloved by the most high God. Wow, how's that for esteem. Take it in, hold it close and stand firm in that concept and this verse for one moment before we move on to All Out. Since we were made in God's likeness, we represent the righteousness in Him. **Isaiah 41:10 -So do not fear, for I am with you; do not be dismayed, for I am your God. I will strengthen you and help you; I will uphold you with my righteous right hand.**

This righteousness is not something we can earn, it is freely given, I love that. Freely given because of a beautiful love story of my God who laid down His life for little ole' me, and yes you. **Romans 3:22 - This righteousness is given through faith in Jesus Christ to all who believe.**

The measure at which you would have to love someone to give-up your life for them, just think about this for a moment. I am asking myself as I write this, who would I love that much and that deep. I can only come-up with a very short list of people who would come close to me dying for, knowing it was the only way for them to live. The love that this takes is astounding and it is indeed making this connection for yourself is huge with understanding your worth. It is what healthy esteem is made-up of, the truth of the lengths to which our God loves us. That he loves us with an intimate, customized to us love. He knows the ins and outs of our thoughts, faults, weaknesses, strengths and chose to die so we would be righteous. This is beauty at its finest, this is a love story that endures the test of time, this is something worth texting.

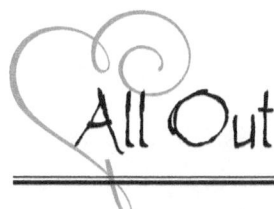

All Out

So interestingly enough, the next chapter of this book and my life as we progress was not nearly as much about sex and attention as it seems most courting experiences are. What was unique to me about my suitor is that sex was not the number one thing on his mind. In this case, it should have been a red flag but for me the thought of someone not being so preoccupied with something that was so all-dominating in my world, it caught my attention. Don't get me wrong, I did marry pregnant so there was sex but it definitely wasn't the focus. Then it quickly became about our sweet precious child not us.

Just want to take a moment and talk about girls who get pregnant before they are married. We as a culture need to love on them so fiercely, support them in entirety. For some reason, once a girl is pregnant in many circles, there is this impression that she has ruined her life and is basically a carrier now for a new life. Now don't get me wrong, I coach girls to wait and have sex until after marriage, I coach about abstaining and being smart if you absolutely can't abstain.

However, if a girl is pregnant and she tells you she is pregnant, please love her ferociously. Don't wait for her to get engaged, make the decision you want her to make, come to you for love - love her immediately, do not pass Go/do not collect $200, love her!

She is wrestling with some of the most challenging esteem issues ever. She most likely feels very guilty, possibly doesn't have a ton of family support and is now connected with some other being who she isn't even sure she wants to be with. As someone who went through teen unwed pregnancy, there is a lot too it, be kind.

Now the sweet girl who arrived shook my world like nothing else. I have never wanted someone protected, happy, loved, everything good. This is what happens when you become a parent. You cease to exist the way you were before and you are now a new person who is seriously dedicated to the survival of this person. If done right, being a parent, changes your entire world. I love my daughter more than I can even explain through words. I was not ready to be a parent and she showed me such grace it makes me teary to even express how good she was to me. When my next child came, I was older I was 25 and much more aware of what it meant to love and protect another person. They both are my entire world and the greatest example of God's miracles in my life, to me.

The point of All Out though is not the great love that I have for my children, although this is core to my being, it is about being completely disconnected to that part of me that God wired for intimacy and touch.

You see Sex Esteem isn't just about unhealthy ways of getting attention, it is also about total denial of who you are and how God made you. God made me to be very passionate, extremely affectionate and in-love with spending time together. To disconnect from how God made you is not healthy either.

During this phase of my life I was all out of touch with the ways God made me to thrive in this particular area called intimacy. Now don't get me wrong, I loved on my children, my friends children in a healthy wonderful way. I gained incredible friendships that have been my anchor and bless me in uncountable ways.

I worked to become a professional who may not always be liked but is generally respected. I studied and studied, achieving my associates, bachelors, and masters without enduring student debt but I allowed myself to get lost in a different way. I had real needs, me not my family but me and I allowed them to be compromised over and over again. I allowed how God made me to be unsupported and muted. This is also a misuse of God's intention. He wants us to be cherished, loved mightily and not settle for anything less.

I knew myself enough to put certain boundaries in place, I would not be one of those women who cheated on her husband. I would not compromise on my integrity, I would dive into all things pure…. children, christian music, girlfriends. Just a note this book is not about marriage, I respect my ex as my children's father way too much to write in detail about that experience, this book is about me and my experience using sex and lack of sex as my esteem indicator. During this phase of my life, I was all out when it came to who God made me in this area.

I believe this verse about my body being a temple and honored that in tangible ways, **1ˢᵗ Corinthians 6: 19-20 - Do you not know that your bodies are temples of the Holy Spirit, who is in you, whom you have received from God? You are not your own; 20 you were bought at a price.** Therefore honor God with your bodies. I took care of my mind, body and spirit and focused on the good continually. I communicated what I thought I was lacking to who I needed to, sought counseling and continued doing what I could do as a Godly wife. I focused on God's stuff, and tried desperately to be ok with suppressing the part of me that was wired for passion.

God had truly changed me, He sanctified me so physical and emotional connection no longer drove my esteem, now He did. I was completely a new self and this was both exciting and free'ing. I trusted God through every high and low, He was my constant when my world was upside down.

This discipline of running to God in times of need is one of the most thankful traits of my life. When the problems or dark shadows come, I run straight to God. There is no other way for me. His loyalty through this time was unsurpassed, the way He used me to pour into others lives and keep our children steady was incredible.

In many ways, God is the best husband that I will ever have and I am tremendously thankful for this truth. He truly made me a new creation without denying the way He wired me, this is true love. **Romans 6:6 - For we know that our old self was crucified with him so that the body ruled by sin might be done away with, that we should no longer be slaves to sin.**

Now don't get me wrong, I had feelings and advances. I worked in corporate america with primarily men for 90% of my career. There were men who implied, straight out asked, recognized my passion expressed through work and wanted it for their own, I did a good job of staying pure. I had three distinct times in my life that I almost succumbed to this old self. These were in the form of thoughts as I never crossed that line, I think when you marry you take an oath and to compromise yourself in anyway to not be united with your husband is Sin, thoughts included but as we know I am not perfect.

Thankfully for my own integrity I never touched another man in an inappropriate way during my marriage. This makes me sleep well every single night by the way. I had a couple really important rules, one I would never stay out late on business trips, drinking was not ok for me, would avoid driving in the car with someone of the opposite sex. These were just a few ways that I found to keep my eyes fixed on Jesus. There were more proactive reminders listed under the Single section of who Sex Esteem is written for.

I do think there is value in walking through the three temptations that I had and the way Jesus helped.

I have worked with some great people and one leader was absolutely incredible when it came to ethics. He was stellar and there was a moment where I thought what if. Then I quickly turned my mind off and focused on the work at hands.

There was another guy who was really fun, just all out silly and I remember calling him once on a sunny day and saying how cool he was and all of a sudden the sun stopped and the rain started coming down so hard. It was like God was saying, stop it, not ok.

Then the last one was during a very difficult part of my life. I had been going to counseling for almost a year, and had a plan for the next chapter of my life. This person reminded me of my value through words and kindness, then he chose to exit when I could have used a friend most.

There was no touch associated with these three encounters but they still impacted my heart and needed to be dealt with. This is a testimony to us really needing to guard our hearts with who we interact with and how we do.

Continually, through ups and downs, the best way for me is to turn my eyes to the most loyal amazing boyfriend, husband, best friend and sovereign God ever. I love how He is always there for me, always. There is nothing that you can't handle with Him by your side. This verse is quoted often but there is a reason for that, **Philippians 4:13 - I can do all this through him who gives me strength.**

Life is messy or can be and when the shifting seas take you in a direction that makes you feel uncertain, whisper this verse to yourself. Remember everything that you have gone through and who you are in Him.

We are not meant to do this walk alone, one of my favorite characteristics of our God is He doesn't just give us the bare minimum to get through life, He makes it sweet. I need to pause for a moment and tell a story, come with me.

Right after I filed for divorce, something I hope you never have to do, I was struggling. The decision to file wasn't why I was struggling, it had been a long time coming and I knew it was the only choice I had left. I was struggling because I wanted God with me even more tangibly than He always had been. Having God as a husband is wonderful because He is the Genesis 1 God but let's face it, not a ton of hugging happens!

So I was visiting Washington state, attending service at a church there I like when I heard a song that I had never heard before. It was Great are you Lord and has so many beautiful lines some of which are, "You give life, you are love, you bring light to the darkness....its your breath in our lungs, so we pour out our praise." This song touched me in a very tangible way, honestly it felt like a giant hug wrapped around me. I became teary and felt God's spirit so alive in me.

Fast forward the next week, I am sitting in my home church in Wisconsin. This beautiful song plays, again I had never heard it and now two weeks in a row, in different states this song plays for me. Again, it feels like a giant hug.

God is incredible. Several times over the last two years, when I have felt unsettled not in my faith but in a tangible request of God, he brings me this song. I have now experienced it at four unrelated churches in four different states, during several prayer meetings and worship nights. There is no rhyme or reason to why it is played other than God knows I need a bit more of Him in a way that feels like a hug. For someone who loves physical touch, this is such a beautiful way that He loves me.

Back in

For anyone who has played team sports and has experienced that feeling of being put "back in", you can relate to this stage of life that I am in. Being given a second chance at love in life motivates me to make it the best possible testimony I can. I want to bring so much glory to God and really just have fun. I think good clean innocent fun is some of the best way to bond with individuals. My esteem comes from the best Yes for God in the moment, not from the world or would be suitors. God is using all of me for His ministry, even the messy parts of my past. I know who I am in Him more every single day.

The misconception about faith is that it is something that we obtain or somewhere that we arrive at. Being Back in is to every single day remind myself that God has me. I may not feel it, I may not understand it but I choose faith, which then leads to joy, which then leads to a Kingdom perspective which then pours into who I am and fills up my esteem. It is a habit like any other.

Six years ago, on my anniversary I bought myself a gift. It is a necklace, quite simple design, from a Christian bookstore that spells Faith on it. This purchase was a commitment from God that He would always be there for me. Even when I felt alone, sad, ugly, hopeless, and not enough. I have worn this necklace every single day since.

Although I don't believe any one thing can hold God, not a church, bumper sticker, or necklace, I will tell you sometimes I just hold this necklace and feel better. The reason is not because of the metal, it is because of time and time again my God coming through. In a life of ups and downs, He has been the one constant. Every single time I run to Him, He is there. When I believe I have nothing to offer, He helps turn my gaze to Him.

I notice when I am not especially feeling high with esteem, if I can get myself busy about the things of Him, all of a sudden I can actually feel who I am again in God and I forget all the insecurities that try to convince me that I am not good enough to serve.

One of the things people tend to call me is an encourager. I am thankful that God has equipped in me an ability to see the best in people. Most people don't know but seeing the best in people and accepting them the way they are is part of being a follower of God.

This verse rings particularly true, **Romans 15:7 - Accept one another, then, just as Christ accepted you, in order to bring praise to God.** Through accepting one another, this means good, bad, ugly, indifferent, etc., we are actually showing the image of God. One of the fantastic characteristics of God is His welcoming us to come be with Him exactly how we are. This means that I don't need to pretty myself up or hide the parts of me that I am self-conscious about. Then that acceptance of who He is comes full circle with our ability to take our focus off of ourselves and instead focus on loving others.

The part that I am just learning about traditionally having your esteem be poured in from others is that it becomes a constant cycle. I love the way one teacher put it, there is a God size hole in all of us and we try to fill it with all sorts of junk, nothing can fill it except Him. This filling-up is continual. Every single day, you chose to fill yourself up with something, what that something is will determine how you feel about your worth.

The surprise to me though is that I really think God wants us to have fun as we are Back in the game, so for instance, play, rest, how you are wired to enjoy life is really part of the process. I have heard all sorts of sermons where they talk about God being portrayed as a kill-joy when in fact He is the one who designed pleasure and fantastic laughter.

The feeling you get when you are in the zone of cooking, gardening, writing, just being. These are all God's melodies. For those of us wired for work primarily or who have lost our identity in sports, school, work, relationships, that truth of just being is incredibly healing.

The trick with being back in is to not allow your mind to wander to past mistakes or future anxieties. Asking yourself is this really important, is it edifying and is it advancing God's glory. I love this verse, **Colossians 3: 1:3 - 1 Since, then, you have been raised with Christ, set your hearts on things above, where Christ is, seated at the right hand of God. 2 Set your minds on things above, not on earthly things. 3 For you died, and your life is now hidden with Christ in God.**

The reason I love this verse is it shows the power we have over our minds and hearts. We are not slaves to the way we feel, instead we have the power to set our minds on things above. Set is an interesting action word. It is full of purpose, being set apart, setting something up high. Setting our hearts on thoughts, ideas and impressions that are higher than temporal concerns shows who we are for eternity. When we are concerned with who we are in eternity, we are less concerned about that muffin top or boy who said he wasn't attracted to us.

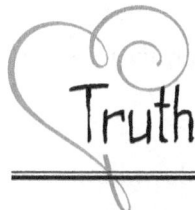# Truth

We've made it. I have been eagerly waiting us to get to this chapter. Truth is how we conquer leaning towards having our esteem in anything other than who we are designed to be.

The key to victory over this area is really in being grounded in the truth. Feelings and truth many times can be enemies. Have you ever had an experience where you really felt offended and all of a sudden you have a different memory or truth of the words said or deeds done?

This is because when we are mixed up by feelings, if we don't take a moment to check ourself in the truth, we will be blurred by mistruths.

The first truth of who we are is illustrated in this verse well, **1ˢᵗ Peter 2:9 - But you are a chosen people, a royal priesthood, a holy nation, God's special possession, that you may declare the praises of him who called you out of darkness into his wonderful light.**

We are a mighty priesthood. This truth is incredibly freeing. We can intercede for ourselves with Christ who dwells in us. This means that the power to change, ask for forgiveness, say no to lust, guilt, shame lies right in our own hands. God already did the hard work of making a way, now we just need to walk in it.

Another mistruth that impacts this area is if we come from a family that didn't provide good direction, support and education in this area.

We need to remember what Kingdom family we are part of, this verse reference is **Ephesians 1:5 - he predestined us for adoption to sonship through Jesus Christ, in accordance with his pleasure and will.** We belong to a family, hand picked into a family. Any missing parts of your upbringing can be healed through this family that you are adopted into.

The last truth that I will leave you with is that we are loved with an unimaginable love. One of our pastors frequently referred to us as beloved, this very quickly became my daughters favorite word for herself. It is such a beautiful illustrative name, beloved. **1ˢᵗ John 3:1-2 - See what great love the Father has lavished on us, that we should be called children of God! And that is what we are! The reason the world does not know us is that it did not know him. 2 Dear friends, now we are children of God, and what we will be has not yet been made known. But we know that when Christ appears, we shall be like him, for we shall see him as he is.**

Whichever phase you may be at, whether a girl just learning about these feelings, a wild woman trying to navigate change, a wife who has become apathetic to passion, or a single trying to pursue the will of God, thank you for listening to my journey. Thank you for understanding these truths and trying to apply them to your life.

By sharing some of my story, we have a pact. I hope to hear about your story. Please share it, there is power in removing the shame, minimizing the sin and shining God's glory as bright as we can. Be encouraged, feel and make good choices.

Girlfriends

It hit me as I was having coffee with my dear girlfriends, there is no way I would be where I am today with my battle with sex esteem without my girlfriends.

Seriously, God has given me the best girlfriends on the planet. When I am not sure what to do, when I want to be silly, when I want to cry, when I want to be quiet, when I need to hike....when I can't pray but need to. It is incredible because for a lot of my life, I haven't been a huge fan of women. They seemed to backstab and talk about such petty things. I now know, that is just some women and generally ones who are trying to hide what is really going on with them.

Once you have had girlfriends who stand by you through thick and thin, pick you up from the fetal position, remind you who you are when your name has been slandered all over the internet, help you decorate for your daughter's party, make sure you have a sparkle in your eye when you talk about someone special...you will never forget them.

Proverbs 18:24 - One who has unreliable friends soon comes to ruin, but there is a friend who sticks closer than a brother.

My girlfriends have been there for me through thick and thin. Ladies often ask me how I can have such deep friendships with so many. Quite simply, I am honestly and unashamedly me and if they can meet

me in that truth, awesome. If not, they head their way and I head my way. I have very little skill or tolerance for small talk. Honestly, I could do completely without it. Living in the midwest where one can always talk about the weather has helped divert my disdain for small talk but it still is there. My girlfriends are so close to me they give me strength when I most need it.

This next verse is especially important to me, **Proverbs 12:26 - The righteous choose their friends carefully, but the way of the wicked leads them astray.** The reason it is important to me is that who we spend time with is a choice. Some of our girlfriends suck the very life out of us, they don't mean to but they are not fillers of our cup. Others are fillers of our cup and we feel recharged by spending time with them. Some lead us into gossip and buying things we can't afford and eating too much when we don't want to. Some know our soft spots and lead us towards righteousness by offering sound counsel. Choosing who you spend time with, when you are weak, strong and in between will determine the choices you make over and over again. Choose wisely.

There have been times when my girlfriends have given me advice and I am sorry to say I haven't followed it. There have also been times when they have given me advice and I have followed it. The point is, people doing life with you makes you live sharp, aware, present and strong. **Proverbs 27:17 - As iron sharpens iron, so one person sharpens another.**

Significant milestones in life serve as excellent pruners of friends. Through many of the most challenging parts of my life, people have decided they can't "deal" with being in my life. This is such a blessing, it proves who is really in the long-haul with you and who isn't. I don't know about you but I only have so much energy and the fewer people who I have to think they are for me, when they really aren't the better. **Proverbs 17:17 - A friend loves at all times, and a brother is born for a time of adversity.** This verse sums up this concept well.

I remember the first time I realized that love from friends was critical for health. After growing up pursuing the affection of the opposite sex, and trying to gain sex esteem, it was wonderful to understand that healthy harmonious platonic relationships are critical. We are stronger together, period.

While this verse generally references marriage, and while I hope someday to have the kind of marriage that it shows, for me at this moment it is the perfect picture of my dear friends and me - whether hiking through the snow or walking on the farm, down the pier, in the mall, this verse shows me when I let someone else in who is trust worthy we yield more than when I fight this fight solo. **Ecclesiastes 4:9-10 - Two are better than one, because they have a good return for their labor: 10 If either of them falls down, one can help the other up. But pity anyone who falls and has no one to help them up.**

My choices haven't always been great with friends, some have really hurt me by showing me their true colors, not giving me the benefit of the doubt and just being overall self-absorbed. With prayer and observation, plus the good old test of time you will know who people really are and if they are for you. **Proverbs 13:20 - Walk with the wise and become wise, for a companion of fools suffers harm.**

Sword – Bible Reference Page

Who is Sex Esteem for? - Romans 8:1, There is no condemnation for those who belong to Christ Jesus.

Who is Sex Esteem for? - Romans 8:28, And we know that in all things God works for the good of those who love him, who have been called according to his purpose.

What are these feelings? - 1 Corinthian 6:17 - But whoever is united with the Lord is one with him in spirit.

What are these feelings? - Genesis 1:27 - So God created mankind in his own image, in the image of God he created them; male and female he created them.

What are these feelings? - Jeremiah 17:9 - The heart is deceitful above all things, and desperately sick; who can understand it?

All In - John 1:12 - Yet to all who did receive him, to those who believed in his name, he gave the right to become children of God.

All In - 1 John 3:20 - For whenever our heart condemns us, God is greater than our heart, and he knows everything.

All In - Isaiah 41:10 -So do not fear, for I am with you; do not be dismayed, for I am your God. I will strengthen you and help you; I will uphold you with my righteous right hand.

All In - Romans 3:22 - This righteousness is given through faith in Jesus Christ to all who believe.

All Out - 1ˢᵗ Corinthians 6: 19-20 - Do you not know that your bodies are temples of the Holy Spirit, who is in you, whom you have received from God? You are not your own; 20 you were bought at a price. Therefore honor God with your bodies.

All Out - Romans 6:6 - For we know that our old self was crucified with him so that the body ruled by sin might be done away with, that we should no longer be slaves to sin.

All Out - Philippians 4:13 - I can do all this through him who gives me strength.

Back In - Romans 15:7 - Accept one another, then, just as Christ accepted you, in order to bring praise to God.

Back In - Colossians 3: 1:3 - 1 Since, then, you have been raised with Christ, set your hearts on things above, where Christ is, seated at the right hand of God. 2 Set your minds on things above, not on earthly things. 3 For you died, and your life is now hidden with Christ in God.

Truth - 1ˢᵗ Peter 2:9 - But you are a chosen people, a royal priesthood, a holy nation, God's special possession, that you may declare the praises of him who called you out of darkness into his wonderful light.

Truth - Ephesians 1:5 - he predestined us for adoption to sonship through Jesus Christ, in accordance with his pleasure and will.

Truth - 1ˢᵗ John 3:1-2 - See what great love the Father has lavished on us, that we should be called children of God! And that is what we are!

The reason the world does not know us is that it did not know him. 2 Dear friends, now we are children of God, and what we will be has not yet been made known. But we know that when Christ appears, we shall be like him, for we shall see him as he is.

Girlfriends - Proverbs 12:26 - The righteous choose their friends carefully, but the way of the wicked leads them astray.

Girlfriends - Proverbs 27:17 - As iron sharpens iron, so one person sharpens another.

Girlfriends - Proverbs 17:17 - A friend loves at all times, and a brother is born for a time of adversity.

Girlfriends - Ecclesiastes 4:9-10 - Two are better than one, because they have a good return for their labor: 10 If either of them falls down, one can help the other up. But pity anyone who falls and has no one to help them up.

Girlfriends - Proverbs 13:20 - Walk with the wise and become wise, for a companion of fools suffers harm.

Girlfriends - Proverbs 18:24 - One who has unreliable friends soon comes to ruin, but there is a friend who sticks closer than a brother.